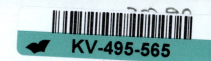
PUBLIC HEALTH IN THE 21ST CENTURY

PUBLIC HEALTH IN THE 21ST CENTURY

Additional books in this series can be found on Nova's website under the Series tab.

Additional E-books in this series can be found on Nova's website under the E-books tab.

BACTERIOLOGY RESEARCH DEVELOPMENTS

Additional books in this series can be found on Nova's website under the Series tab.

Additional E-books in this series can be found on Nova's website under the E-books tab.

CLOSTRIDUM DIFFICILE-ASSOCIATED DIARRHEA

HIDEAKI KATO

Novinka
Nova Biomedical Books
New York

Library of Congress Cataloging-in-Publication Data

Available upon Request
ISBN: 978-1-61728-278-2

Published by Nova Science Publishers, Inc. ✦ New York

Contents

Preface

Clostridium difficile is a gram-positive anaerobic, spore-forming bacterium involved in antibiotic-associated diarrhea and colitis, which is developed after administration of antibiotics. *C. difficile* is nosocomially transmissible via hospital staff and contaminated environmental surface as well between patients. *C. difficile* infection results in a broad spectrum of disease ranging from mild diarrhea to severe life-threatening condition. Colonic injury and inflammation are caused by the two types of toxins: toxin A and B produced by the bacteria. Diagnosis of *C. difficile*-associated diarrhea is due to identification of one/both of the two toxins or the bacterial antigen (glutamate dehydrogenase) and propagation of *C. difficile* in stools from the patients. The colonoscopic picture reveals multiple mucosa nodules with raised, yellowish white plaques (pseudomembranes) with normal intervening mucosa. With progression, the pseudomembranes can coalesce, forming confluent plaques that may slough. So far, *C. difficile* had been classified into more than 100 PCR ribotypes. Epidemiology and difference of pathogenecity of each type have not been fully elucidated. Recently, the incidence and severity of *C. difficile*-associated diarrhea have increased significantly. These changes are associated with the emergence of a hypervirulent epidemic strains of *C. difficile* (North American pulsed-field gel electrophoresis type 1 (NAP1)/PCR ribotype 027). Discontinuation of the offending antibiotics is an important first step in the treatment of *C. difficile*-associated diarrhea. Oral administration of vancomycin or metronidazol is the standard and promising therapy and can achieve favorable response in 97% of the cases. Recurrence is observed in approximately 15% of treated cases. Judicious use of antimicrobials and infection control measures, such as cohorting patients with symptom, use of chlorhexadine in hand washing and use of environmental disinfectant, prevent the development of *C. difficile* infection.

Chapter I

Introduction

Clostridium difficile is a gram-positive, an anaerobic, spore-forming, rod and is the most common cause of infectious gastrointestinal disease among hospitalized patients. Antibiotic-associated diarrhea is important and increasingly frequent complications of antibiotic therapy. Antibiotic-associated diarrhea that is caused by *Clostridium difficile* is called as *C. difficile*-associated diarrhea (CDAD) and accounts for 15~20% of all the cases of antibiotic diarrhea (Fekety, 1997). *C. difficile*-associated infection (CDI) causes a wide spectrum of clinical manifestations ranging from an asymptomatic carrier state to fulminant colitis with toxic megacolon. So far, *C. difficile* has been classified into more than 150 polymerase chain reaction (PCR) ribotypes by a study group in the United Kingdom (Stubbs *et al.*, 1999). Recently, *C. difficile* BI type, determined by restriction endonuclease analysis (REA); NAP1 type, determined by pulsed-field gel electrophoresis (PFGE); and PCR ribotype 027 (BI/NAP1/027) have been reported to cause an increasing incidence of *C. difficile* diarrhea and more severe disease than other types in North America and Europe (Warny *et al.*, 2005), (McDonald *et al.*, 2005). Here we describe the pathogenesis and recent findings of *C. difficile*-associated disease and review the literature.

Chapter II

Historical Perspective

The original report of pseudomembranous lesion in the intestinal tract appeared in the Bulletin of John's Hopkins in 1893 (Ros *et al.*, 1996). The case was a 22-year-old patient who underwent gastric surgery and subsequently developed severe diarrhea. The patient was died and autopsy revealed "diphtheritic membranes" in the intestine. Pseudomembranous colitis was a rare condition until the introduction of antibiotics, when it became relatively common adverse effect of treatment with tetracycline and chloramphenicol. The association between antibiotic use and pseudomembranous colitis was suggested as early as 1952 by Reiner *et al.* (1952) and widely accepted 1974 when Tedesco *et al.* prospectively studied the colonic sequelae of clindamycin use (Ros *et al.*, 1996). Tedesco and colleagues investigated 200 patients treated with clindamycin and found that 41 patients (21%) developed diarrhea, and 20 (50%) out of the 41 patients had pseudomenbranes detected by endoscopy. In the early period, *Staphylococcus aureus* is considered to the etiologic agent of pseudomembranous colitis because the bacteria was the major nosocomial pathogen and was identified in stool culture with high frequency. One of the most important findings reported by Tedesco *et al.* was that the absence of *S. aureus* in pseudomembranuos colitis, although the bacteria was relatively easy to grow in selective cultures. *C. difficile* was first recognized as a component of the normal intestinal flora of newborn infants by Hall and O'Toole in 1935 (Hall and Duffett, 1935). At that time, the organism was named as *"Bacillus difficilis"* due to its nature of "difficult" propagation in culture. Bartlett *et al.* subsequently identified *C. difficile* as the offending pathogen (Bartlett *et al.*, 1978). These investigators were further able to reveal that *C. difficile* toxin rather than a viral or direct bacterial process mediated antibiotic-associated colitis.

Chapter III

Genetic Organization

The full genome sequence of *C. diffcile* was firstly determined in "630" strain Sebaihia *et al.* (2006) in "630" strain which is PCR-ribotype 012 and was a multi-drug-resistant isolate from a patient with PMC at a hospital in Zurich in 1982. The full genome length of 630 strain was revealed to a 4.29 Mb chromosome with a mosaic of potential mobile genetic elements, antibiotic resistance genes and virulence determinants. Stabler *et al.* developed a microarray based on 630 strain sequence (Stabler *et al.*, 2006) and investigated 75 diverse isolates comprising hypervirulent, toxin-variable, and animal strains, and found four distinct, statistically supported clusters. One was a hypervirulent cluster and another toxin A negative toxin B positive clone. Only 19.7% of the wider spectrum of genes analysed were shared by all strains, and they concluded that the organisms can indeed readily undergo genetic exchange. Eleven % of the DNA was related to mobile elements, including antimicrobial resistance. Several genetic islands were found relating to virulence, adhesion, antibiotic resistance, motility and enteric metabolism. There was no spore forming genes (i.e. its sporulation mechanisms are quite different from known sequences). Furthermore, the ABC transported system was located on conjugative transposons and may be relevant to the trigger factors of proton pump inhibitors and quinolones.

Chapter IV

Epidemiology

Antibiotics-associated diarrhea and colitis are important and increasing frequent complications of antibiotic therapy. The incidence of diarrhea during antimicrobials chemotherapy ranges from 5 to 30%, on a variety of factors, including the definition of diarrhea and the type of antibiotics (Bartlett, 1992; Tedesco, 1975). While these occur most often in hospitals and nursing homes, they also occur in the community. Between 10 and 25% of all cases of antibiotic-associated diarrhea in industrialized countries are ascribed to *C. difficile*, but this is based on data for hospitalized patients (Viscidi *et al.*, 1981; Surawicz *et al.*, 1989a).

In healthy infant, relatively high rate of carriage (2%~60%) in the feces is reported. Donta & Myers reported that 10.5% of 105 healthy newborns surveyed were culture positive and that 28/51 (51%) of babies on a neonatal intensive care unit had toxin positive stools. (Donta and Myers, 1982) . A scandinavian study found *C. difficile* in 60% of 218 healthy neonates, peaking at a rate of 64% carriage in the age group 1-8 months (Holst *et al.*, 1981). el-Mohandes *et al.* reported that 50 preterm babies housed in an intensive care facility over the first 34 days of life, sampling at weekly intervals, and 15% culture-positive during week 1, rising to 33% at week 2 and stayed until the end of observation (el-Mohandes *et al.*, 1993) . Larson *et al.* reported that 2%~52% of infant were positive for *C. difficile*, but the carriage rate of *C. difficile* vary between wards in the same hospital (Larson *et al.*, 1982). Acquisition of the organism by the neonate is commonly considered to be from the hospital environment (Bolton *et al.*, 1984; Sherertz and Sarubbi, 1982), although there are some studies suggesting maternal transmission (Donta and Myers, 1982). Despite the fact that rate of carriage of *C. difficile* is high, symptoms associates with *C. difficile* is rarely seen. Why infants remain unaffected by the toxins is explained by immaturity of toxin receptor of the intestine in infants which is susceptible for disease progression but the precise mechanism is still under discussion.

It is well recognized that healthy adults can carry *C. difficile* without any symptoms and intestinal carriage rates of *C. difficile* in healthy adults vary considerably. Previously, surveys on healthy adults including a large number of samples had been carried out and shown that intestinal colonization of healthy adults by *C. difficile*, colonization rates ranges from 0 to 17.5% (Aronsson *et al.*, 1985; Nakamura *et al.*, 1981; Viscidi *et al.*, 1981; Wilson *et al.*, 1982). Kato *et al.* (2001) investigated 1234 healthy adults who were not exposed antimicrobials for the preceding 4 weeks and found that colonization rates of toxigenic and non-toxigenic *C. difficile* ranged from 4.2 to 15.3% depending on the surveyed groups. Fekety & Shah reported that the feces of about 5% of healthy adults are colonized by toxigenic *C. difficile* (Fekety and Shah, 1993). A Swedish study of 594 volunteers found a carriage rate of 1.9% and Phillips & Rogers (1981) reported a 2% of isolation rate in 100 random stool samples that are negative for other pathogens. Many factors may influence the results of such studies. For instance, the fact that whether antibiotics is not taken (at least a month) before sampling, the size of the study, the ethnic origin of the study group, and the culture methods employed are important factors (Brazier, 1998).

Whether gut carriage is a permanent or temporary state is under discussion. A longitudinal study using PCR methods to detect low numbers of the bacteria could give an answer this issue. Carriage of *C. difficile* in the healthy adults gut might be usually transient and some isolates would be just "passing through" at the time of sampling (Brazier, 1998). Kato *et al.* investigated 139 healthy adults from two study groups (university students and company employees) by stool culture at an interval of 3 months for 1 year (Ozaki *et al.*, 2004). They found that 18 individuals (12.9%) were positive for *C. difficile* and frequency of isolation of *C. difficile* in each individual were once in 10 subjects, twice in 3, three times in 2, and four times in 3. Thus in the 3 (2.2%) subjects *C. difficile* had been isolated for one-year study period. It seems that colonization by *C. difficile* strains is transient in many cases but there also exists healthy individuals colonized persistently by *C. difficile*.

Chapter V

Classification

Several typing schemes have been developed to determine the relatedness of strains of *C. difficile* associated with infection, including serotyping (Delmee *et al.*, 1985; Toma *et al.*, 1988), immunoblotting (Heard *et al.*, 1986), arbitrarily primed PCR (Barbut *et al.*, 1993b), pulsed-field gel electrophoresis (PFGE; Collier *et al.*, 1996), PCR ribotyping (Cartwright *et al.*, 1995; Gurtler, 1993), and *slpA* typing method (Kato *et al.*, 2005). With so many typing methods for *C. difficile* described in the literature, it is not clear if one method will ever become established as the universal typing scheme. Obviously, some form of standardization would greatly enhance surveillance and advance our knowledge of the global epidemiology of CDI. There are, however, attempts to establish some form of standardization in the nomenclature ascribed to strains typed by the various methods (Brazier *et al.*, 1994).

Serogroup

Serogrouping by slide agglutination with rabbit antisera, together with the protein profiles obtained by polyacrylamide gel electrophoresis (PAGE), enables the differentiation of 14 serogroups, designated by capital letters (A, B, C, D, F, G, I, K, S1, S2, S3, S4, and X) (Delmee *et al.*, 1986; Toma *et al.*, 1988). In serogroup A, another 20 subgroups

(subgroups A1 to A20) can be distinguished by PAGE (Delmee *et al.*, 1986).

Toxinotyping

Based on variability of pathogenicity locus (PaLoc), *C. difficile* isolates were classified into 10 toxinotypes and those were named using Roman numerals I to X (Rupnik *et al.*, 1998). Toxinotypes correlate well with the types obtained by two other typing schemes (serogrouping and PFGE typing). This method for the typing of *C. difficile* toxin genes could be easily performed in routine raboratory practice, where it could be used to detect and characterize variant strains and to monitor their prevalence. So far, 24 toxinotypes had been reported.

PCR Ribotyping

PCR ribotyping has been reported to provide a discriminatory, reproducible, and simple alternative to other typing method. It is based on differences in profiles generated with PCR primers designed to amplify the 16S-23S rRNA gene intergenic spacer region (Stubbs *et al.*, 1999). This technique has a number of advantages over other methods; specifically, PCR ribotyping has been shown to be more discriminatory than arbitrarily primed PCR and serotyping and is quicker and simpler than PFGE. PCR ribotyping has one further advantage over PFGE, since some isolates of *C. difficile* have excessive endogenous nuclease activity that render them untypeable by PFGE. Stubbs *et al.* showed that *C. difficile* isolates has been classified into 116 PCR ribotypes (Stubbs *et al.*, 1999). To date, more than 150 PCR-ribotypes had been reported.

REA

Kuijper *et al.* (1987) used whole-cell DNA REA with *HindIII* in a study which suggested cross-infection between two patients in the same room. A study applied REA to 205 isolates from 106 patients and demonstrated 55 distinct patterns, indicating a high degree of strain diversity in their population (Samore *et al.*, 1994). Those indicated that REA is a highly discriminatory and reproducible method, but is technically requiring and rather laborious.

Arbitrarily Primer PCR (AP-PCR)

AP-PCR is based on nonspeciric random amplifications by PCR of the bacterial chromosom using a short primer under low-stringency conditions. It permits the detection of polymorphism without prior knowledge of the target nucleotide sequence. Chachaty *et al.* applied AP-PCR to 30 unrelated isolates and they were classified into 20 distinct types (Chachaty *et al.*, 1994). However, the results were poorly reproducible, a criticism often leveled at methods using arbitrary primers.

Pulsed-field Gel Electrophoresis (PFGE)

PFGE differs from conventional agarose electrophoresis in that it can separate very large DNA fragments by alternating the direction of the current between two sets of electrodes at an obtuse angle. This allow the whole chromosome to be analysed after digestion with rare cutting restriction endonucleases, such as *SmaI*, *KspI*, *SacII* or *NruI*, which produce up to ten RFLPs per strain.

Surface Layer Protein a (slpA) Typing

This method based on the amplification of *slpA* gene of *C. difficile* by PCR and the amplified product is sequenced (Kato *et al.*, 2005). Sequence typing has the advantage of enabling easy comparison of typing result among multiple laboratories without exchanging reference strains as is required in typing systems which depend on banding-pattern analysis. This technique has highly discrimination power and PCR-ribotype smz is classified into 3 *slpA* types using *slpA* typing method base on 1 point-mutation within *slpA* gene.

Chapter VI

Risk Factors

Risk factors for development of CDI are listed Table 1. A large number of risk factors for development of CDI had been reported. Almost all the patients with CDI are prescribed with antibiotics and anticancer drugs before development the disease. It might be better to deal with the two factors "trigger factor" than "risk factor" because those two agents are absolutely imperative for the development of CDI. Hospitalization is the second important factors for development of CDI. Reasons for this that CDI is the leading cause of infectious diarrhea among hospitalized patients and is also rarely seen among outpatients. Even if the individuals developed CDI as outpatients, they usually have the history of hospitalization within a few months before the onset. Advanced age (>65)(Bates *et al.*, 1990; Gifford and Kirkland, 2006; Brown *et al.*, 1990), prolonged hospital stay (Guyot *et al.*, 2000), concurrent hospitalization with carriers or patients with active infection (Clabots *et al.*, 1992), severity of underlying disease (Gerding *et al.*, 1986), renal failure (Dial *et al.*, 2004) Aseeri *et al.*, 2008), respiratory tract infection (Lai *et al.*, 1997), gastrointestinal procedure (Brown *et al.*, 1990)), and immunosuppressive treatment (Arslan *et al.*, 2007) are well known as the risk factors of CDI.

Table 1. Risk factors for development of CDI

Antibiotics*	Hospitalization
Second generation cephalosporin	Prolonged hospital stay
Third generation cephalosporin	Advanced age (>65)
Clindamycin	Lung cancer
Moxifloxacin	Neutropenia
Clarythromycin	Bone marrow and peripheral blood stem cell transplantation
Norfloxacin	Intensive care residence
Ciprofloxacin	Gastrointestinal procedure
Penicilline	Respiratory tract infection
Cefotaxime	Number of receipt of antimicrobials (≥3)
Cefuroxime	Duration of exposure to second-generation cephalosporin
Erythromycin	Admission within 3 months
Ceftazidime	Renal failure
Metronidazole	Tube feeding
Aminoglycoside	Administration of interleukin-2
Lincomycin+aminoglycoside	Severity of underlying disease
Ampicillin	Presence of another case in same ward
Ampicillin+amoxicillin	Graft versus host disease grade 3-4
Anticancer drugs	Enema
Taxane	Gastrointestinal stimulant
Methorexate	More than ten antibiotic days
Immunosupressant	
Antiacids	
Proton pump inhibitor	

* All antibiotics except for vancomycin is potentially associated with development of CDI.

Antimicrobials

The use of antimicrobial agents, particularly multiple treatment courses and/or broad-spectrum agents including clindamycin, cephalosporins, and quinolones, are the most common risk factor for developing CDI. Almost all antimicrobials could be the risk factor for developing CDI. Antimicrobials disturb the normal intestinal flora, which acts as a colonization barrier in a normal state, protects against *C. difficile*. Destruction of intestinal flora allows the proliferation of *C. difficile* in the intestine. It is noteworthy that some kinds of antimicrobials seem to be strongly linked to outbreak of CDI. In the case of outbreak of CDI in the diverse hospital in the U.S. (Samore *et al.*, 1997), *C. difficile* strains resistant to clindamycin had been identified. *C. difficile* strains resistant to clindamycin clearly harbored a propensity to cause epidemics because in outbreaks caused by clindamycin-resistant *C. difficile*, there was rapid resolution of the epidemic with restriction of the use of clindamycin (Climo *et al.*, 1998; Pear *et al.*, 1994). There are some case reports that describe *C. difficile*-associated colitis after use of clarithromycin, for example, for otitis in an infant and following the eradication of *H. pyroli* in an adult (Braegger and Nadal, 1994) ; Archimandritis *et al.*, 1998). Quinolon is also a well-known risk factor for CDI. In the study of 1980's, it is reported that quinolones such as ciprofloxacin and norfloxacin are relatively inactive against *C. difficile* (Delmee and Avesani, 1986; Chow *et al.*, 1985), while ciprofloxacin and other oral quinolones are active against many intestinal bacteria and are highly concentrated in the stool. Therefore, it is plausible microbilogically that quinolones predispose to CDI by eradicating normal gut flora and allowing toxigenic strains of *C. difficile* to proliferate. In fact, a possible relationship between quinolone use and CDI has been described in several case reports and case-control studies (Bates *et al.*, 1990; Cain and O'Connor, 1990; Ehrenpreis *et al.*, 1990; McFarland *et al.*, 1995).

Whether preoperative prophylactic antibiotics were a risk factor for CDI is or not has controversies. The selection of *C. difficile* in fecal flora and the anecdotal occurrence of CDI following even a single dose of antibiotics are well reported (Block *et al.*, 1985; Freiman *et al.*,1989; Bombassaro *et al.*, 2001), while prophylactic antibiotics had not been shown to be a specific risk factor for developing CDI (Teasley *et al.*, 1983; Palmore *et al.*, 2005).

Proton Pump Inhibitors

Recently, association between proton pump inhibitors and development of CDI among hospitalized patients are reported (Aseeri *et al.*, 2008) but the association between the agents and the development of CDI have controversies. A potential mechanism for facilitation of development of CDI by proton pump inhibitors is that inhibition of gastric acidity resulting in the loss of a defense mechanism against ingested spores and bacteria. Having higher gastric pH than normal facilitates the survival of *C. difficile* spores and their toxins while in the vegetative state by affecting leukocyte function (Dial *et al.*, 2005; Wilson *et al.*, 1985). An increased risk of CDI with acid suppression therapy could thus arise from undigested vegetative cells being allowed to pass into the distal gastrointestinal tract. Even so, several reports indicated that contribution of PPI for development of *C. difficile*-associated diarrhea seems to be low. It should be minded that clinicians should avoid that continuation of subscription of PPIs during subsequent hospital admissions without evaluating the necessity of continuing such therapy.

Chapter VII

Pathogenecity

Pathogenic strains of *C. difficile* typically produce two high-molecular-weight toxins that share a considerable degree of homology and function but vary in respect to target cell specificity. Toxin A, the enterotoxin, causes fluid secretion in the ileal loop assay, and toxin B is a potent cytotoxin to many different eukaryotic cell lines. Isolates that produce neither toxin are non pathogenic. Toxins A and B are encoded in a part of the genome designated the pathogenesity locus. Along with the gene for a porin protein (*tcdE*), the pathogenecity locus includes two regulatory genes, *tcdC* and *tcdD*. A loss of function mutation of the *tcdC* gene in NAP1/027 is thought to be responsible for its marked upregulation of toxin production. A third toxin, called binary toxin, is expressed by only a minority of *C. difficile* strains and is encoded in a separate part of the genome. The epidemic strain expression binary toxin but its role, if any, in causing or exacerbating CDI is unknown. Homologous to the iota toxin of *Clostridium perfringens*, it is an ADP ribosyltransferase that also causes actin distegration. Binary toxin causes fluid secretion, but no evident epithelial damage. in rabbit intestine. Once antibiotic therapy has made the bowel susceptible to infection, colonization by *C. difficile* occurs by the oral-fecal route. *C. difficile* forms heat-resistant spores that persist in the environment for months or years. Infection results from oral ingestion of these spores, which serrvive the acid environment of the stomach and convert to vegetative forms in the colon. Antibiotic therapy is the key factor that alters the colonic flora and allows *C. difficile* to flourish. The colon is home to more than 500 species of bacteria, and normal stool may contain as many as 10^{12} bacteria per gram. The disruption of the normal bacteria flora in the colon, colonization with *C. difficile*, and the release of toxins that cause mucosal damage and inflammation (Kelly *et al.*, 1994). Research has shown that patients usually unexposed to *C. diffcile* throughout their hospitalizations and that antibiotic use promotes the acquisition of *C. dificile*. The outcome of acquisition, which may be colonization or infection with *C. difficile*, is thought to be determined primarily by patient factors including advanced age and severity of underlying illness, which may compromise the ability to mount an immune response against the bacteria (Bates *et al.*, 1990).

Although initially thought to be nonpathogenic, toxin A-negative, toxin B-positive strain have been recovered from numerous patients with classic manifestations of *C. difficile* diarrhea and gave been responsible for outbreaks of diarrhea and colitis in hospitals in Canada, Polan, the U.K., France, Japan, and The Netherland (van den Berg *et al.*, 2004).

The factors that influence the severity of the symptom are now better understood. For instance, the age of the patient is an important factor; most of the severe cases are seen in patients over 65 or 70 years. The level of the immune response such as circulating IgG or local IgA against toxin A also demonstrated to be the key factor for development and severity of *C. diffcile*-associated diseases. Patients with severe symptoms have significantly lower serum- and feces-specific antibody levels than those with milder symptoms (Warny *et al.*, 1994). Moreover, a serum antibody response to toxin A during an initial episode of CDI is associated with protection against recurrence (Kyne *et al.*, 2001). It has also been shown that, after colonization of a patient by *C. difficile*, there is an association between a systemic response to toxin A, as evidenced by increases serum levels of IgG antibody against toxin A, and asymptomatic carriage of *C. dffffcile* (Kyne *et al.*, 2000).

Chapter VIII

Symptoms

Symptoms generally start during antibiotics therapy but can be delayed by several weeks to months. The typical symptoms include profuse watery diarrhea together with cramping abdominal pains, sometimes associates with temperatures (over 39℃), volume depletion and high leucocyte count. Fever and leucocytosis are common but nonspecific findings. Leukocytosis is found in the stool in about 50% of the cases, but do not distinguish *C. difficile*-associated diarrhea from other inflammatory diseases (Burke *et al.*, 1988). Obstination secondary to ileus may characterize the toxic form of the disease and mimic colonic pseudo-obstruction, volvulus and toxic megacolon. Therefore, absence of diarrhea should not be considered atypical or preclude the diagnosis (Medich *et al.*, 1992; Lipsett *et al.*, 1994). Historically, threat of fulminant *C. difficile* colitis ranges from 1% to 3% (Kelly and LaMont, 1998) (Figure 1). Toxic megacolon is a well recognized, potentially fatal complication of colitis, and first recognized as a clinical entity by Marschal *et al.* in 1950. It is defined as segmental or total colonic distenstion of >6 cm in the presence of acute colitis and sign of systemic toxicity (Marshak and Lester, 1950). Fatal complication that account for death due to pseudomembranous colitis are toxic heat failure, shock due to volume depletion, toxic, megacolon, colonic wall perforation and massive lower gastrointestinal hemorrhage (Totten *et al.*, 1978).

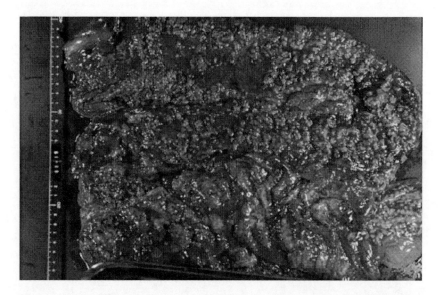

Figure 1. Gross appearance of the resected colon specimen from a 72-year-old woman with severe pseudomembranous colitis, developed after antibiotic therapy. The specimens shows multiple, widely distributed pseudomenbranes in the entire colon.

Chapter IX

Diagnosis

Laboratory Tests

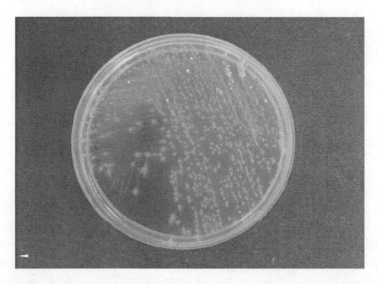

Figure 2. Propagation of *C. difficile* CCFA. Colony of *C. difficile*. Small round white-yellowish colony is seen in CCFA.

The definitive diagnosis made by detection of the organism, its toxins, other cellular antigens, and most recently toxin-specific genes. It has been recommended that patients who developed diarrhea more than 3 days after admission should be tested for *C. difficile* as the possible infectious etiology for their symptom (Bauer *et al.*, 2001) since *C. difficile* is the most commonly recognized cause of diarrhea in hospitalized patients. The first choice of diagnosing *C. difficile* infection is immunoassays for detecting toxins and antigens of *C. difficile*. Numerous rapid tests are commercially available, and many have been clinically evaluated (Barbut *et al.*, 2003; Turgeon *et al.*, 2003). The clinical significance of toxin A-negative/toxin B-positive variants (Massey *et al.*, 2003) warrants use of immunoassay for both. Although those rapid tests can serve the result within several hours, those are woefully inadequate in terms of diagnostic sensitivity. The studies showed the sensitivity of the rapid immunoassys to detect *C. difficile* below 60% when compared with PCR detection of toxins A and B genes (Morelli *et al.*, 2004; van den Berg *et al.*, 2005). Traditionally, the tissue culture cytotoxicity assay detecting the presence of *C. difficile* cytotoxin (toxin B) is stool filtrate is considered to be the "gold standard" for diagnosis because of high sensitivity (Vanpoucke *et al.*, 2001; Barbut *et al.*, 1993a)(100-1000 fold more sensitive than EIA) and specificity (99%-100%) (Wilkins and Lyerly, 2003; Delmee, 2001). The cytotoxic culture requires a tissue culture facility and required 48 h to produce the result. Stool culture for detection of the *C. difficile* is the most sensitive method to detecting the organism (Figure 2). However, culture of *C. difficile* is labour-intensive and results are not available at least 72-96 hours. Furthermore, stool culture has the potential for detecting nontoxigenic strain of *C. difficile*. However, stool culture has the advantage of enabling strain typing for investigation of an outbreak. How can we increase the use of *C. difficile* culture in microbiology laboratories? From the standpoint of treatment, culture and identification of toxigenic *C. difficile* alone is not a satisfactory approach, because results are obtained too slow to be any use for rapidly progressive *C. difficile* clinical illness in some patients. A practical algorithm would seem to be for laboratories to continue performing immunoassays for toxins along with stool culture, since their specificity of immunoassays is high. If the initial test result is negative, the toxigenic culture and PCR could either be reflexively performed when suspicion of *C. difficile* is high.

Endoscopy

Colonoscopy can detect the characteristic adherent white or yellowish white plaques that vary in diameter from 2 to 10 mm (Figure 3a). In patients with severe disease, the plaque may coalescence to cover large areas of the mucosa (Figure 3b). In almost the cases, the pseudomembrane is observed in left side of the colon, however, approximately 10 percent of cases, colitis is confined to the more proximal colon therefore may be missed during sigmoidoscopy. In fulminant colitis, colonoscopy should not be performed due to the risk of perforation, however, proctoscopy with minimal insufflation of air may be a useful diagnostic tool (Kawamoto *et al.*, 1999). Pathologically, mucosal necrosis, polymorphonuclear cells deep to the lumen propria without deeper layer destruction, and thrombosed vessels or abscess are seen in biopsied specimen from pseudomembranous mucosa (Wald *et al.*, 1980).

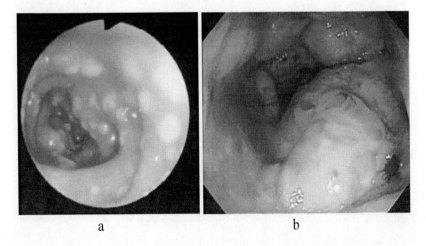

a   b

Figure 3. Endoscopic findings of pseudomembranous colitis (PMC). a. Picture shows characteristics yellow plaques representing pseudomembranes. b. Endoscopic finding of severe case of PMC. Pseudomembrane completely involves the visible segments of the colon circumferentially.

Radiology

Plain radiolographic findings in *C. difficile* associated diarrhea vary depending of the severity and extent of disease (Figure 4). Boland *et al.* (1994) reported radiolographic abnormalities in 32% of 152 hospitalized patients with positive stool toxin assay. Colonic ileus was found in 32% of patients, follows small bowel ileus (20%), nodular haustra thickening (18%), and ascites 7%. Futhermore, trhum-printing (unusual, wide transverse bands associated with thickening of the haustral folds) and gaseous distension of the colon are also seen.

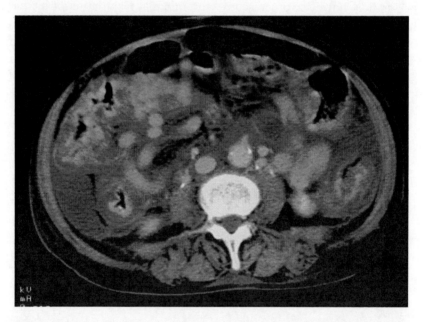

Figure 4. CT finding of PMC. Wall thickness of the colon wall and ascites are seen.

CT has been used for the evaluation of acute abdominal diseases and has proved helpful in the diagnosis of *Clostridium difficile*-associated diseases (Figure 5). Wall thickening, such as low-attenuation mural thickening corresponding to mucosal and submucosal edema, and ascites are seen in the cases of *Clostridium difficile*-associated diseases. Fishman *et al.* reported that the wall thickness of the colon was more severe (average 14.7mm, in many cases the wall thickness was over 20 mm) than that of ulcerative colitis (average 7.8 mm) and Crohn's disease (average 13 mm).

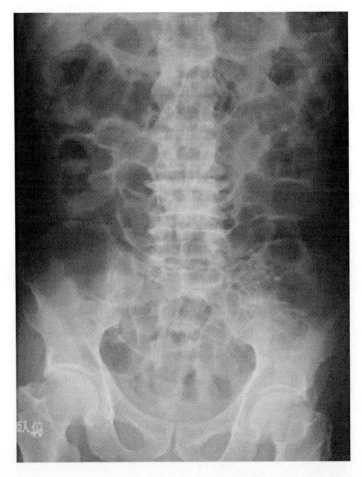

Figure 5. Abdominal X-ray of toxic megacolon due to PMC. The film shows dilatation of transverse colon (>8 cm), thickening and obscuring of hastra, and retention of gas in the small intestine, indicating paralytic ileus are seen.

"Accordion sign", which is first described Fishman *et al.* (1991), is seen when orally administered contrast material becomes trapped between markedly thickened haustral folds, giving the appearance of alternating bands of high attenuating (contrast material) and low attenuation (edematous haustra). This accordion sign is suggestive of pseudomembranous colitis, although it is usually seen only in advanced cases. Its appearance varies depending on the degree of edema of the haustral fold and the amount of contrast material trapped between the folds (Kawamoto *et al.*, 1999). In the 1990, "According sign" is reported to a specific CT finding of peudomembranous colitis (Ros *et al.*, 1996; Fishman et al., 1991),. Macari and Bosniak (1999) reported that 15 patients with "accordion sign" on CT were retrospectively investigated and reported that only 4 out of the 15 patients were indentified *C. difficile* in their stool and different causes were documented in the remaining 11 paitents. Therefore, they concluded that "accordion sign" is suggestive of pseudomombranous colitis but not specific for it and is a nonspecific finding in patients with colonic edema. Nowadays the use of CT imaging in the diagnosis of pseudomambranous colitis has limitation but this modality is noninvasive, easy, rapid.

Chapter X

BIII/NAP1/027 Strain

Increased numbers of patients requiring colectomy alerted a hospital in Montreal, Quebec, Canada in 2002 to the possibility of CDI with higher severity, mortality and relapse rate (Loo *et al.*, 2005). Over the next two years, several investigations were performed: rate of CDI were ~28/1000 admissions (five times the natural average of 1997) and 30-day attributed mortality rates of 6.9%, these being 0.8-2% in 1997. Strain typing of isolates from involved Quebec hospitals revealed that 129 of 157 isolates tested (82.2%) were of a single strain, NAP1/027 (North American PFGE type I/ribotype 027(Loo *et al.*, 2005). Between 2004 and 2005 it was estimated that over 14 000 patients has been affected in the province of Quevec, with high mortality and relapse rate. A similar situation to that in Canada had emerged in the USA, with the Centers for Disease Control and Prevention (CDC) showing rates has doubled between 1996 and 2003 from 31 to 61 cases per 100 000. McDonald et al (McDonald *et al.*, 2005) performed strain typing on 187 isolates from eight institutions in six different states that had seen higher than normal rates of CDI in the U.S. The 027 strain is widely distributes in North America and has been reported from Great Britain, The Netherlands, and Belgium (Joseph *et al.*, 2005; Kuijper *et al.*, 2006; MacCannell *et al.*, 2006; Smith, 2005).

Although the NAPI/027 strain was previously a minor strain in isolates collections, it was the predominant strain in this epidemic. Warny *et al.*(2005) quantified toxin production by the NAP1/027 strain and found it to produce over 16 and 23 times as much toxin A and toxin

B respectively as historic isolates (toxinotypoe 0) of *C. difficile* (Noren, 2005). The NAP1/027 strain carries an 18 base pair deletion in the *tcdC* gene, a natural inhibitor of toxin expression that may account for its increased toxin production and virulence.

Chapter XI

Treatment

When the diagnosis is made soon after the onset of diarrhea, and antibiotics is stopped, the *C. difficile*-associated diarrhea seems to be self-limiting with no mortality, thus, early diagnosis and disease-specific intervention can be life-saving (Burke *et al.*, 1988). Studies have shown that resolution of diarrhea occurs in 15~23% of patients when removal of the causative antibiotic is the only the intervention employed (Olson *et al.*, 1994; Fekety, 1997). For moderate or severe condition of *C. difficile* diarrhea or patients in whom offending antibiotics cannot be discontinued, antimicrobial therapy is required. Oral metronidazole therapy (250 mg 4 times daily or 500 mg twice daily) given for 10-14 days is recommended as the initial treatment (Gerding *et al.*, 1995); Fekety, 1997). Vancomycin (125 mg orally 4 times daily for 10-14 days) is the recommended second line therapy (Gerding *et al.*, 1995; Fekety, 1989,1997). Vancomycin given orally has very minimal absorption and achieves stool level more than 1000 µg/mL of stool, which exceeds the MIC by at least 1000-fold (Fekety, 1997; Tedesco *et al.*, 1978). Both metronidazole and vancomycin therapy had been demonstrated to have the similar efficacy rate of 90~97% (Olson *et al.*, 1994). Given the higher cost of oral vancomycin therapy and concern about selection for vancomycin-resistant enterococci, metronidazole is preferred as the initial agent of choice (Gerding *et al.*, 1995; Fekety, 1997). Vancomycin should be reserved for patients with contraindications or intolerance to metronidazole or for those who failed to respond to metronidazole after five days of treatment (Bartlett, 2002). Clinical response rates for patients treated with oral bacitracin have been 10~20% lower than those treated with vancomycin and the agent is considered to a third line option after metronidazole and vancomycin (Novak *et al.*, 1976). In addition to specific antimicrobial therapy, supportive therapy with hydration and correction of electrolyte abnormalities is important in patients with *C. difficile*-associated diarrhea. The use of antidiarrheal agents and opiates for management of CDI should be avoided in order to prevent masking of symptoms, retention of toxin-laden secretions in the colon, and the development of severe colitis (Novak *et al.*, 1976; Kato *et al.*, 2007, 2008). Response to CDI therapy can be assessed initially by resolution of fever typically within the first two days, followed by resolution of diarrhea, which is seen within the first two to four days. Treatment should be continued for seven to 10 days, with therapeutic failures not assessed until treatment has been given for at least five days (Bartlett, 2002).

Despite initial response rates of more than 90%, recurrence of *C. difficile*-associated diarrhea occurs in about 5%-20% of patients after treatment with either metronidazole or vancomycin (Zimmerman *et al.*, 1997; Barbut *et al.*, 2000; Fekety, 1997). Possible reasons for a relapse include a failure to eradicate the organism from the colon or reinfection from the environment, both of which may be related to the formation of antibiotic-resistant *C. dificile* spores. After an initial relapse, the risk of further recurrences has been reported to be as high as 65%, with a median of 3 relapses and a range of 2 to 9 (Fekety *et al.*, 1997). Recurrences occurred at a median of 8 days, with range of 1 to 42 days (Fekety *et al.*, 1997). For patients with multiple relapses, tapered and pulsed antibiotic therapy with vancomycin has been used. Tapered dose regimen of vancomycin is that 125 mg every 6 hours for 7 days, followed by every 12 hours, then daily, then every other day (each for 7 days; total 28 days), pulsed dose regimen of vancomycin is that 125 to 500 mg every 2 to 3 days for 3 weeks, and taper plus pulsed dose regimen is that start with a tapering dose of 28 days, followed by 21 days of pulsed dosing (Oldfield, 2004). Because low levels of IgG antitoxin A have been associated with recurrent disease, some authors have used IVIG with success in patients with multiple relapses and low levels of specific antibody (Leung *et al.*, 1991).

Adjunctive therapy with probiotic agents such as *Saccaromyces boulardii* (Surawicz *et al.*, 1989b, 2000; McFarland *et al.*, 1994) and

Lactobacillus GG (Gorbach *et al.*, 1987) has also found to be effective in the management of a relatively small number of patients with recurrent *C. difficile*-associated diarrhea.

Chapter XII

Prevention

The main concern with *C. difficile* is that, once hospitalized patients get diarrhea, they very rapidly contaminate their environment with spores that are very resistant and may persist for months, thus creating the potential for a hospital outbreak. (Kelly and LaMont, 1998). Prevention of nosocomial transmission of *C. difficile* depends on careful attention to hand-washing, isolation and barrier precautions, and cleaning of the physical environment throughout the duration of symptomatic disease. Good hand-washing practice (with either a disinfectant or soap) and glove use had been shown to be effective in preventing *C. difficile* transmission. The use of isolation techniques (enteric isolation, private rooms, and cohorting of infected patients) has been employed for outbreak control with varied success. These measures are based on the premise that patients with active CDI are the primary source for spread of disease within the institution. Environmental contamination has been linked to spread of *C. difficile* via a contaminated commode chair, a nursery baby bath, and contaminated electric rectal thermometer handles. The risk of transmission via contaminated endoscopes appears to be low if scopes are glutaraldehyde immersion for as little as 5 minutes. In vitro testing of glutaraldehyde preparations also indicated that exposure of *C. difficile* spores to 2% alkaline glutaraldehyde for 12 minutes is sporicidal. Disinfection is effective in reducing the number of *C. difficile*-positive cultures from the environment. A study showed unbuffered hypochlorite (500 ppm available chlorine) to disinfect the ward environment during a small *C. difficile* outbreak and reduced the ward contamination rate from 31.4% to 16.5% of samples sites. Limitation or restriction of use of agents also found to be associated with increased CDI rates, such as clindamycin, cephalosporins, and ampicilline is an intuitively attractive approach to reduction of cases.

References

Archimandritis, A., Souyioultzis, S., Katsorida, M., and Tzivras, M. (1998). *Clostridium difficile* colitis associated with a 'triple' regimen, containing clarithromycin and metronidazole, to eradicate Helicobacter pylori. *J. Intern. Med. 243*, 251-3.

Aronsson, B., Mollby, R., and Nord, C. E. (1985). Antimicrobial agents and *Clostridium difficile* in acute enteric disease: epidemiological data from Sweden, 1980-1982. *J. Infect. Dis. 151*, 476-81.

Arslan, H., Inci, E. K., Azap, O. K., Karakayali, H., Torgay, A., and Haberal, M. (2007). Etiologic agents of diarrhea in solid organ recipients. *Transpl. Infect. Dis. 9*, 270-5.

Aseeri, M., Schroeder, T., Kramer, J., and Zackula, R. (2008). Gastric acid suppression by proton pump inhibitors as a risk factor for *Clostridium difficile*-associated diarrhea in hospitalized patients. *Am. J. Gastroenterol. 103*, 2308-13.

Barbut, F., Delmee, M., Brazier, J. S., Petit, J. C., Poxton, I. R., Rupnik, M., Lalande, V., Schneider, C., Mastrantonio, P., Alonso, R., Kuipjer, E., and Tvede, M. (2003). A European survey of diagnostic methods and testing protocols for *Clostridium difficile*. *Clin. Microbiol. Infect. 9*, 989-96.

Barbut, F., Kajzer, C., Planas, N., and Petit, J. C. (1993a). Comparison of three enzyme immunoassays, a cytotoxicity assay, and toxigenic culture for diagnosis of *Clostridium difficile*-associated diarrhea. *J. Clin. Microbiol. 31*, 963-7.

Barbut, F., Mario, N., Frottier, J., and Petit, J. C. (1993b). Use of the arbitrary primer polymerase chain reaction for investigating an outbreak of *Clostridium difficile*-associated diarrhea in AIDS patients. *Eur. J. Clin. Microbiol. Infect. Dis. 12*, 794-5.

Barbut, F., Richard, A., Hamadi, K., Chomette, V., Burghoffer, B., and Petit, J. C. (2000). Epidemiology of recurrences or reinfections of *Clostridium difficile*-associated diarrhea. *J. Clin. Microbiol. 38*, 2386-8.

Bartlett, J. G. (1992). Antibiotic-associated diarrhea. *Clin. Infect. Dis. 15*, 573-81.

Bartlett, J. G. (2002). Clinical practice. Antibiotic-associated diarrhea. *N. Engl. J. Med. 346*, 334-9.

Bartlett, J. G., Chang, T. W., Gurwith, M., Gorbach, S. L., and Onderdonk, A. B. (1978). Antibiotic-associated pseudomembranous colitis due to toxin-producing clostridia. *N. Engl. J. Med. 298*, 531-4.

Bates, C. J., Wilcox, M. H., Spencer, R. C., and Harris, D. M. (1990). Ciprofloxacin and *Clostridium difficile* infection. *Lancet. 336*, 1193.

Bauer, T. M., Lalvani, A., Fehrenbach, J., Steffen, I., Aponte, J. J., Segovia, R., Vila, J., Philippczik, G., Steinbruckner, B., Frei, R., Bowler, I., and Kist, M. (2001). Derivation and validation of guidelines for stool cultures for enteropathogenic bacteria other than *Clostridium difficile* in hospitalized adults. *JAMA. 285*, 313-9.

Block, B. S., Mercer, L. J., Ismail, M. A., and Moawad, A. H. (1985). *Clostridium difficile*-associated diarrhea follows perioperative prophylaxis with cefoxitin. *Am. J. Obstet. Gynecol. 153*, 835-8.

Boland, G. W., Lee, M. J., Cats, A., and Mueller, P. R. (1994). Pseudomembranous colitis: diagnostic sensitivity of the abdominal plain radiograph. *Clin. Radiol. 49*, 473-5.

Bolton, R. P., Tait, S. K., Dear, P. R., and Losowsky, M. S. (1984). Asymptomatic neonatal colonisation by *Clostridium difficile*. *Arch. Dis. Child. 59*, 466-72.

Bombassaro, A. M., Wetmore, S. J., and John, M. A. (2001). *Clostridium difficile* colitis following antibiotic prophylaxis for dental procedures. *J. Can. Dent. Assoc 67*, 20-2.

Braegger, C. P., and Nadal, D. (1994). Clarithromycin and pseudomembranous enterocolitis. *Lancet. 343*, 241-2.

Brazier, J. S. (1998). The epidemiology and typing of *Clostridium difficile*. *J. Antimicrob. Chemother. 41* Suppl C, 47-57.

Brazier, J. S., Delmee, M., Tabaqchali, S., Hill, L. R., Mulligan, M. E., and Riley, T. V. (1994). Proposed unified nomenclature for *Clostridium difficile* typing. *Lancet. 343*, 1578-9.

Brown, E., Talbot, G. H., Axelrod, P., Provencher, M., and Hoegg, C. (1990). Risk factors for *Clostridium difficile* toxin-associated diarrhea. *Infect. Control Hosp. Epidemiol. 11*, 283-90.

Burke, G. W., Wilson, M. E., and Mehrez, I. O. (1988). Absence of diarrhea in toxic megacolon complicating *Clostridium difficile* pseudomembranous colitis. *Am. J. Gastroenterol. 83*, 304-7.

Cain, D. B., and O'Connor, M. E. (1990). Pseudomembranous colitis associated with ciprofloxacin. *Lancet.* 336, 946.

Cartwright, C. P., Stock, F., Beekmann, S. E., Williams, E. C., and Gill, V. J. (1995). PCR amplification of rRNA intergenic spacer regions as a method for epidemiologic typing of *Clostridium difficile. J. Clin. Microbiol. 33*, 184-7.

Chachaty, E., Saulnier, P., Martin, A., Mario, N., and Andremont, A. (1994). Comparison of ribotyping, pulsed-field gel electrophoresis and random amplified polymorphic DNA for typing *Clostridium difficile* strains. *FEMS Microbiol. Lett. 122*, 61-8.

Chow, A. W., Cheng, N., and Bartlett, K. H. (1985). In vitro susceptibility of *Clostridium difficile* to new beta-lactam and quinolone antibiotics. *Antimicrob. Agents Chemother. 28*, 842-4.

Clabots, C. R., Johnson, S., Olson, M. M., Peterson, L. R., and Gerding, D. N. (1992). Acquisition of *Clostridium difficile* by hospitalized patients: evidence for colonized new admissions as a source of infection. *J. Infect. Dis. 166*, 561-7.

Climo, M. W., Israel, D. S., Wong, E. S., Williams, D., Coudron, P., and Markowitz, S. M. (1998). Hospital-wide restriction of clindamycin: effect on the incidence of Clostridium difficile-associated diarrhea and cost. *Ann. Intern. Med. 128*, 989-95.

Collier, M. C., Stock, F., DeGirolami, P. C., Samore, M. H., and Cartwright, C. P. (1996). Comparison of PCR-based approaches to molecular epidemiologic analysis of *Clostridium difficile. J. Clin. Microbiol. 34*, 1153-7.

Delmee, M. (2001). Laboratory diagnosis of *Clostridium difficile* disease. *Clin. Microbiol. Infect. 7*, 411-6.

Delmee, M., and Avesani, V. (1986). Comparative in vitro activity of seven quinolones against 100 clinical isolates of *Clostridium difficile*. *Antimicrob. Agents Chemother. 29*, 374-5.

Delmee, M., Homel, M., and Wauters, G. (1985). Serogrouping of *Clostridium difficile* strains by slide agglutination. *J. Clin. Microbiol. 21*, 323-7.

Delmee, M., Laroche, Y., Avesani, V., and Cornelis, G. (1986). Comparison of serogrouping and polyacrylamide gel electrophoresis for typing *Clostridium difficile*. *J. Clin. Microbiol. 24*, 991-4.

Dial, S., Alrasadi, K., Manoukian, C., Huang, A., and Menzies, D. (2004). Risk of *Clostridium difficile* diarrhea among hospital inpatients prescribed proton pump inhibitors: cohort and case-control studies. *CMAJ. 171*, 33-8.

Dial, S., Delaney, J. A., Barkun, A. N., and Suissa, S. (2005). Use of gastric acid-suppressive agents and the risk of community-acquired *Clostridium difficile*-associated disease. *JAMA. 294*, 2989-95.

Donta, S. T., and Myers, M. G. (1982). *Clostridium difficile* toxin in asymptomatic neonates. *J. Pediatr. 100*, 431-4.

Ehrenpreis, E. D., Lievens, M. W., and Craig, R. M. (1990). *Clostridium difficile*-associated diarrhea after norfloxacin. *J. Clin. Gastroenterol. 12*, 188-9.

el-Mohandes, A. E., Keiser, J. F., Refat, M., and Jackson, B. J. (1993). Prevalence and toxigenicity of *Clostridium difficile* isolates in fecal microflora of preterm infants in the intensive care nursery. *Biol. Neonate. 63*, 225-9.

Fekety, R. (1997). Guidelines for the diagnosis and management of *Clostridium difficile*-associated diarrhea and colitis. American College of Gastroenterology, Practice Parameters Committee. *Am. J. Gastroenterol. 92*, 739-50.

Fekety, R., McFarland, L. V., Surawicz, C. M., Greenberg, R. N., Elmer, G. W., and Mulligan, M. E. (1997). Recurrent *Clostridium difficile* diarrhea: characteristics of and risk factors for patients enrolled in a prospective, randomized, double-blinded trial. *Clin. Infect. Dis. 24*, 324-33.

Fekety, R., and Shah, A. B. (1993). Diagnosis and treatment of *Clostridium difficile* colitis. *JAMA. 269*, 71-5.

Fekety, R., Silva, J., Kauffman, C., Buggy, B., and Deery, H. G. (1989). Treatment of antibiotic-associated *Clostridium difficile* colitis with oral vancomycin: comparison of two dosage regimens. *Am. J. Med.* *86*, 15-9.

Fishman, E. K., Kavuru, M., Jones, B., Kuhlman, J. E., Merine, D. S., Lillimoe, K. D., and Siegelman, S. S. (1991). Pseudomembranous colitis: CT evaluation of 26 cases. *Radiology. 180*, 57-60.

Freiman, J. P., Graham, D. J., and Green, L. (1989). Pseudomembranous colitis associated with single-dose cephalosporin prophylaxis. *JAMA. 262*, 902.

Gerding, D. N., Johnson, S., Peterson, L. R., Mulligan, M. E., and Silva, J., Jr. (1995). *Clostridium difficile*-associated diarrhea and colitis. *Infect. Control Hosp. Epidemiol. 16*, 459-77.

Gerding, D. N., Olson, M. M., Peterson, L. R., Teasley, D. G., Gebhard, R. L., Schwartz, M. L., and Lee, J. T., Jr. (1986). *Clostridium difficile*-associated diarrhea and colitis in adults. A prospective case-controlled epidemiologic study. *Arch. Intern. Med. 146*, 95-100.

Gifford, A. H., and Kirkland, K. B. (2006). Risk factors for *Clostridium difficile*-associated diarrhea on an adult hematology-oncology ward. *Eur. J. Clin. Microbiol. Infect. Dis. 25*, 751-5.

Gorbach, S. L., Chang, T. W., and Goldin, B. (1987). Successful treatment of relapsing *Clostridium difficile* colitis with Lactobacillus GG. *Lancet. 2*, 1519.

Gurtler, V. (1993). Typing of *Clostridium difficile* strains by PCR-amplification of variable length 16S-23S rDNA spacer regions. *J. Gen. Microbiol. 139*, 3089-97.

Guyot, A., Rawlins, M. D., and Barrett, S. P. (2000). Clarithromycin appears to be linked with *Clostridium difficile*-associated diarrhoea in the elderly. *J. Antimicrob. Chemother. 46*, 642-3.

Hall, I. C., and Duffett, N. D. (1935). The Identification of von Hibler's "Bacillus VI" as Bacillus carnis (Klein). *J. Bacteriol. 29*, 269-91.

Heard, S. R., Rasburn, B., Matthews, R. C., and Tabaqchali, S. (1986). Immunoblotting to demonstrate antigenic and immunogenic differences among nine standard strains of *Clostridium difficile*. *J. Clin. Microbiol. 24*, 384-7.

Holst, E., Helin, I., and Mardh, P. A. (1981). Recovery of *Clostridium difficile* from children. *Scand. J. Infect. Dis. 13*, 41-5.

Joseph, R., Demeyer, D., Vanrenterghem, D., van den Berg, R., Kuijper, E., and Delmee, M. (2005). First isolation of *Clostridium difficile*

PCR ribotype 027, toxinotype III in Belgium. *Euro Surveill. 10,* E051020 4.

Kato, H., Iwashima, Y., Nakamura, M., Nakamura, A., and Ueda, R. (2008). Inappropriate use of loperamide worsens *Clostridium difficile*-associated diarrhoea. *J. Hosp. Infect. 70,* 194-5.

Kato, H., Kita, H., Karasawa, T., Maegawa, T., Koino, Y., Takakuwa, H., Saikai, T., Kobayashi, K., Yamagishi, T., and Nakamura, S. (2001). Colonisation and transmission of *Clostridium difficile* in healthy individuals examined by PCR ribotyping and pulsed-field gel electrophoresis. *J. Med. Microbiol. 50,* 720-7.

Kato, H., Nakamura, M., and Nakamura, A. (2007). A case of toxic megacolon secondary to *Clostridium difficile*-associated diarrhea worsened after administration of an antimotility agent and molecular analysis of recovered isolates. *J. Gastroenterol. 42,* 507-8.

Kato, H., Yokoyama, T., and Arakawa, Y. (2005). Typing by sequencing the *slpA* gene of *Clostridium difficile* strains causing multiple outbreaks in Japan. *J. Med. Microbiol. 54,* 167-71.

Kawamoto, S., Horton, K. M., and Fishman, E. K. (1999). Pseudomembranous colitis: spectrum of imaging findings with clinical and pathologic correlation. *Radiographics. 19,* 887-97.

Kelly, C. P., and LaMont, J. T. (1998). *Clostridium difficile* infection. *Annu. Rev. Med. 49,* 375-90.

Kelly, C. P., Pothoulakis, C., and LaMont, J. T. (1994). *Clostridium difficile* colitis. *N. Engl. J. Med. 330,* 257-62.

Kuijper, E. J., Oudbier, J. H., Stuifbergen, W. N., Jansz, A., and Zanen, H. C. (1987). Application of whole-cell DNA restriction endonuclease profiles to the epidemiology of *Clostridium difficile*-induced diarrhea. *J. Clin. Microbiol. 25,* 751-3.

Kuijper, E. J., van den Berg, R. J., Debast, S., Visser, C. E., Veenendaal, D., Troelstra, A., van der Kooi, T., van den Hof, S., and Notermans, D. W. (2006). *Clostridium difficile* ribotype 027, toxinotype III, the Netherlands. *Emerg. Infect. Dis. 12,* 827-30.

Kyne, L., Warny, M., Qamar, A., and Kelly, C. P. (2000). Asymptomatic carriage of *Clostridium difficile* and serum levels of IgG antibody against toxin A. *N. Engl. J. Med. 342,* 390-7.

Kyne, L., Warny, M., Qamar, A., and Kelly, C. P. (2001). Association between antibody response to toxin A and protection against recurrent *Clostridium difficile* diarrhoea. *Lancet. 357,* 189-93.

Lai, K. K., Melvin, Z. S., Menard, M. J., Kotilainen, H. R., and Baker, S. (1997). *Clostridium difficile*-associated diarrhea: epidemiology, risk factors, and infection control. *Infect. Control Hosp. Epidemiol. 18*, 628-32.

Larson, H. E., Barclay, F. E., Honour, P., and Hill, I. D. (1982). Epidemiology of *Clostridium difficile* in infants. *J. Infect. Dis. 146*, 727-33.

Leung, D. Y., Kelly, C. P., Boguniewicz, M., Pothoulakis, C., LaMont, J. T., and Flores, A. (1991). Treatment with intravenously administered gamma globulin of chronic relapsing colitis induced by *Clostridium difficile* toxin. *J. Pediatr. 118*, 633-7.

Lipsett, P. A., Samantaray, D. K., Tam, M. L., Bartlett, J. G., and Lillemoe, K. D. (1994). Pseudomembranous colitis: a surgical disease? *Surgery. 116*, 491-6.

Loo, V. G., Poirier, L., Miller, M. A., Oughton, M., Libman, M. D., Michaud, S., Bourgault, A. M., Nguyen, T., Frenette, C., Kelly, M., Vibien, A., Brassard, P., Fenn, S., Dewar, K., Hudson, T. J., Horn, R., Rene, P., Monczak, Y., and Dascal, A. (2005). A predominantly clonal multi-institutional outbreak of *Clostridium difficile*-associated diarrhea with high morbidity and mortality. *N. Engl. J. Med. 353*, 2442-9.

Macari, M., and Bosniak, M. A. (1999). Delayed CT to evaluate renal masses incidentally discovered at contrast-enhanced CT: demonstration of vascularity with deenhancement. *Radiology. 213*, 674-80.

MacCannell, D. R., Louie, T. J., Gregson, D. B., Laverdiere, M., Labbe, A. C., Laing, F., and Henwick, S. (2006). Molecular analysis of *Clostridium difficile* PCR ribotype 027 isolates from Eastern and Western Canada. *J. Clin. Microbiol. 44*, 2147-52.

Marshak, R. H., and Lester, L. J. (1950). Megacolon a complication of ulcerative colitis. *Gastroenterology. 16*, 768-72.

Massey, V., Gregson, D. B., Chagla, A. H., Storey, M., John, M. A., and Hussain, Z. (2003). Clinical usefulness of components of the Triage immunoassay, enzyme immunoassay for toxins A and B, and cytotoxin B tissue culture assay for the diagnosis of *Clostridium difficile* diarrhea. *Am. J. Clin. Pathol. 119*, 45-9.

McDonald, L. C., Killgore, G. E., Thompson, A., Owens, R. C., Jr., Kazakova, S. V., Sambol, S. P., Johnson, S., and Gerding, D. N.

(2005). An epidemic, toxin gene-variant strain of *Clostridium difficile*. *N. Engl. J. Med. 353*, 2433-41.

McFarland, L. V., Bauwens, J. E., Melcher, S. A., Surawicz, C. M., Greenberg, R. N., and Elmer, G. W. (1995). Ciprofloxacin-associated *Clostridium difficile* disease. *Lancet. 346*, 977-8.

McFarland, L. V., Surawicz, C. M., Greenberg, R. N., Fekety, R., Elmer, G. W., Moyer, K. A., Melcher, S. A., Bowen, K. E., Cox, J. L., Noorani, Z., and et al. (1994). A randomized placebo-controlled trial of Saccharomyces boulardii in combination with standard antibiotics for *Clostridium difficile* disease. *JAMA. 271*, 1913-8.

Medich, D. S., Lee, K. K., Simmons, R. L., Grubbs, P. E., Yang, H. C., and Showalter, D. P. (1992). Laparotomy for fulminant pseudomembranous colitis. *Arch. Surg. 127*, 847-52; discussion 852-3.

Morelli, M. S., Rouster, S. D., Giannella, R. A., and Sherman, K. E. (2004). Clinical application of polymerase chain reaction to diagnose *Clostridium difficile* in hospitalized patients with diarrhea. *Clin. Gastroenterol. Hepatol. 2*, 669-74.

Nakamura, S., Mikawa, M., Nakashio, S., Takabatake, M., Okado, I., Yamakawa, K., Serikawa, T., Okumura, S., and Nishida, S. (1981). Isolation of *Clostridium difficile* from the feces and the antibody in sera of young and elderly adults. *Microbiol. Immunol. 25*, 345-51.

Noren, T. (2005). Outbreak from a high-toxin intruder: *Clostridium difficile*. *Lancet. 366*, 1053-4.

Novak, E., Lee, J. G., Seckman, C. E., Phillips, J. P., and DiSanto, A. R. (1976). Unfavorable effect of atropine-diphenoxylate (Lomotil) therapy in lincomycin-caused diarrhea. *JAMA. 235*, 1451-4.

Oldfield, E. C., 3rd (2004). *Clostridium difficile*-associated diarrhea: risk factors, diagnostic methods, and treatment. *Rev. Gastroenterol. Disord. 4,* 186-95.

Olson, M. M., Shanholtzer, C. J., Lee, J. T., Jr., and Gerding, D. N. (1994). Ten years of prospective *Clostridium difficile*-associated disease surveillance and treatment at the Minneapolis VA Medical Center, 1982-1991. *Infect. Control Hosp. Epidemiol. 15*, 371-81.

Ozaki, E., Kato, H., Kita, H., Karasawa, T., Maegawa, T., Koino, Y., Matsumoto, K., Takada, T., Nomoto, K., Tanaka, R., and Nakamura, S. (2004). *Clostridium difficile* colonization in healthy adults:

transient colonization and correlation with enterococcal colonization. *J. Med. Microbiol. 53*, 167-72.

Palmore, T. N., Sohn, S., Malak, S. F., Eagan, J., and Sepkowitz, K. A. (2005). Risk factors for acquisition of *Clostridium difficile*-associated diarrhea among outpatients at a cancer hospital. *Infect. Control. Hosp. Epidemiol. 26*, 680-4.

Pear, S. M., Williamson, T. H., Bettin, K. M., Gerding, D. N., and Galgiani, J. N. (1994). Decrease in nosocomial *Clostridium difficile*-associated diarrhea by restricting clindamycin use. *Ann. Intern. Med. 120*, 272-7.

Phillips, K. D., and Rogers, P. A. (1981). Rapid detection and presumptive identification of *Clostridium difficile* by p-cresol production on a selective medium. *J. Clin. Pathol. 34*, 642-4.

Reiner, L., Schlesinger, M. J., and Miller, G. M. (1952). Pseudomembranous colitis following aureomycin and chloramphenicol. *AMA Arch. Pathol. 54*, 39-67.

Ros, P. R., Buetow, P. C., Pantograg-Brown, L., Forsmark, C. E., and Sobin, L. H. (1996). Pseudomembranous colitis. *Radiology. 198*, 1-9.

Rupnik, M., Avesani, V., Janc, M., von Eichel-Streiber, C., and Delmee, M. (1998). A novel toxinotyping scheme and correlation of toxinotypes with serogroups of *Clostridium difficile* isolates. *J. Clin. Microbiol. 36*, 2240-7.

Samore, M., Killgore, G., Johnson, S., Goodman, R., Shim, J., Venkataraman, L., Sambol, S., DeGirolami, P., Tenover, F., Arbeit, R., and Gerding, D. (1997). Multicenter typing comparison of sporadic and outbreak *Clostridium difficile* isolates from geographically diverse hospitals. *J. Infect. Dis. 176*, 1233-8.

Samore, M. H., Bettin, K. M., DeGirolami, P. C., Clabots, C. R., Gerding, D. N., and Karchmer, A. W. (1994). Wide diversity of *Clostridium difficile* types at a tertiary referral hospital. *J. Infect. Dis. 170*, 615-21.

Sebaihia, M., Wren, B.W., Mullany, P., Fairweather, N.F., Minton, N., Stabler, R., Thomson, N.R., Roberts, A.P., Cerdeño-Tárraga, A.M., Wang ,H., Holden, M.T., Wright, A., Churcher, C., Quail, M.A., Baker, S., Bason, N., Brooks, K., Chillingworth, T., Cronin, A., Davis, P., Dowd, L., Fraser, A., Feltwell, T., Hance, Z., Holroyd, S., Jagels, K., Moule, S., Mungall, K., Price, C., Rabbinowitsch, E.,

Sharp, S., Simmonds, M., Stevens, K., Unwin, L., Whithead, S., Dupuy, B., Dougan, G., Barrell, B., Parkhill, J. (2006) The multidrug-resistant human pathogen *Clostridium difficile* has a highly mobile, mosaic genome. *Nat. Genet.;38*:779-86.

Sherertz, R. J., and Sarubbi, F. A. (1982). The prevalence of *Clostridium difficile* and toxin in a nursery population: a comparison between patients with necrotizing enterocolitis and an asymptomatic group. *J. Pediatr. 100*, 435-9.

Smith, A. (2005). Outbreak of *Clostridium difficile* infection in an English hospital linked to hypertoxin-producing strains in Canada and the US. *Euro Surveill. 10*, E050630 2.

Stabler, R. A., Gerding, D. N., Songer, J. G., Drudy, D., Brazier, J. S., Trinh, H. T., Witney, A. A., Hinds, J., and Wren, B. W. (2006). Comparative phylogenomics of *Clostridium difficile* reveals clade specificity and microevolution of hypervirulent strains. *J. Bacteriol. 188*, 7297-305.

Stubbs, S. L., Brazier, J. S., O'Neill, G. L., and Duerden, B. I. (1999). PCR targeted to the 16S-23S rRNA gene intergenic spacer region of *Clostridium difficile* and construction of a library consisting of 116 different PCR ribotypes. *J. Clin. Microbiol. 37*, 461-3.

Surawicz, C. M., Elmer, G. W., Speelman, P., McFarland, L. V., Chinn, J., and van Belle, G. (1989a). Prevention of antibiotic-associated diarrhea by Saccharomyces boulardii: a prospective study. *Gastroenterology. 96*, 981-8.

Surawicz, C. M., McFarland, L. V., Elmer, G., and Chinn, J. (1989b). Treatment of recurrent *Clostridium difficile* colitis with vancomycin and Saccharomyces boulardii. *Am. J. Gastroenterol. 84*, 1285-7.

Surawicz, C. M., McFarland, L. V., Greenberg, R. N., Rubin, M., Fekety, R., Mulligan, M. E., Garcia, R. J., Brandmarker, S., Bowen, K., Borjal, D., and Elmer, G. W. (2000). The search for a better treatment for recurrent *Clostridium difficile* disease: use of high-dose vancomycin combined with Saccharomyces boulardii. *Clin. Infect. Dis. 31*, 1012-7.

Teasley, D. G., Gerding, D. N., Olson, M. M., Peterson, L. R., Gebhard, R. L., Schwartz, M. J., and Lee, J. T., Jr. (1983). Prospective randomised trial of metronidazole versus vancomycin for *Clostridium-difficile*-associated diarrhoea and colitis. *Lancet. 2*, 1043-6.

Tedesco, F., Markham, R., Gurwith, M., Christie, D., and Bartlett, J. G. (1978). Oral vancomycin for antibiotic-associated pseudomembranous colitis. *Lancet. 2*, 226-8.

Tedesco, F. J. (1975). Ampicillin-associated diarrhea--A prospective study. *Am. J. Dig. Dis. 20*, 295-7.

Toma, S., Lesiak, G., Magus, M., Lo, H. L., and Delmee, M. (1988). Serotyping of *Clostridium difficile. J. Clin. Microbiol. 26*, 426-8.

Totten, M. A., Gregg, J. A., Fremont-Smith, P., and Legg, M. (1978). Clinical and pathological spectrum of antibiotic-associated colitis. *Am. J. Gastroenterol. 69*, 311-9.

Turgeon, D. K., Novicki, T. J., Quick, J., Carlson, L., Miller, P., Ulness, B., Cent, A., Ashley, R., Larson, A., Coyle, M., Limaye, A. P., Cookson, B. T., and Fritsche, T. R. (2003). Six rapid tests for direct detection of *Clostridium difficile* and its toxins in fecal samples compared with the fibroblast cytotoxicity assay. *J. Clin. Microbiol. 41*, 667-70.

van den Berg, R. J., Bruijnesteijn van Coppenraet, L. S., Gerritsen, H. J., Endtz, H. P., van der Vorm, E. R., and Kuijper, E. J. (2005). Prospective multicenter evaluation of a new immunoassay and real-time PCR for rapid diagnosis of *Clostridium difficile*-associated diarrhea in hospitalized patients. *J. Clin. Microbiol. 43*, 5338-40.

van den Berg, R. J., Claas, E. C., Oyib, D. H., Klaassen, C. H., Dijkshoorn, L., Brazier, J. S., and Kuijper, E. J. (2004). Characterization of toxin A-negative, toxin B-positive *Clostridium difficile* isolates from outbreaks in different countries by amplified fragment length polymorphism and PCR ribotyping. *J. Clin. Microbiol. 42*, 1035-41.

Vanpoucke, H., De Baere, T., Claeys, G., Vaneechoutte, M., and Verschraegen, G. (2001). Evaluation of six commercial assays for the rapid detection of *Clostridium difficile* toxin and/or antigen in stool specimens. *Clin. Microbiol. Infect. 7*, 55-64.

Viscidi, R., Willey, S., and Bartlett, J. G. (1981). Isolation rates and toxigenic potential of *Clostridium difficile* isolates from various patient populations. *Gastroenterology. 81*, 5-9.

Wald, A., Mendelow, H., and Bartlett, J. G. (1980). Non-antibiotic-associated pseudomembranous colitis due to toxin-producing Clostridia. *Ann. Intern. Med. 92*, 798-9.

Warny, M., Pepin, J., Fang, A., Killgore, G., Thompson, A., Brazier, J., Frost, E., and McDonald, L. C. (2005). Toxin production by an emerging strain of *Clostridium difficile* associated with outbreaks of severe disease in North America and Europe. *Lancet. 366*, 1079-84.

Warny, M., Vaerman, J. P., Avesani, V., and Delmee, M. (1994). Human antibody response to *Clostridium difficile* toxin A in relation to clinical course of infection. *Infect. Immun. 62*, 384-9.

Wilkins, T. D., and Lyerly, D. M. (2003). Clostridium difficile testing: after 20 years, still challenging. *J. Clin. Microbiol. 41*, 531-4.

Wilson, K. H., Sheagren, J. N., and Freter, R. (1985). Population dynamics of ingested *Clostridium difficile* in the gastrointestinal tract of the Syrian hamster. *J. Infect. Dis. 151*, 355-61.

Wilson, K. H., Silva, J., and Fekety, F. R. (1982). Fluorescent-antibody test for detection of *Clostridium difficile* in stool specimens. *J. Clin. Microbiol. 16*, 464-8.

Zimmerman, M. J., Bak, A., and Sutherland, L. R. (1997). Review article: treatment of *Clostridium difficile* infection. *Aliment. Pharmacol. Ther. 11*, 1003-12.

Index